# PROSTATE CANCER, WHAT I DID TO MAKE IT UNDETECTABLE IN 15 MONTHS

## By Stanley E. Rocklin, Ph.D.

# ACKNOWLEDGMENTS

I want to thank my Facebook friends who, after I put out a call for some ideas on what to name this book, answered my call and gave me good ideas. I was able to cobble together some of the ideas given me to the present title. I promised if one friend came up with the winner, I'd name her/him here. Since each one contributed in a measure, I'd like to name them all. The list might be minus a name or two as I will ask them who wants to be left off the list. Those whose names appear below gave their assent by their not objecting to be listed:

Nita Ornelas

Sue Pecaut Stark

Jerome Puttler

Denise Bassford Cote

Vera House

Betty Mermelstein

# DEDICATION

I want to dedicate this book to my wife, Marlene Rocklin, who helped me edit it, but most important, she gave me the encouragement to stay on my cancer-killer diet and constantly expressed her admiration for my tenacity in  never cheating on it!

*Well, almost never* 

# CHAPTER ONE
## You've got cancer, Stan

My urologist, a medical doctor, my wife Marlene and I sit down in one of the doctor's examining rooms and he tells me that the latest biopsy shows that I have what's known as slow-growing prostate cancer. He shows me photo of the a laboratory slide showing an enlarged view of some of my prostate tissue.

He tells me that 80 percent of 80 year old men in the USA have this form of prostate cancer.

I must forewarn you, I am starting this book out with a funny quip. We look at the slide and I comment that what I am seeing looks like a cat. I point out an ear, mouth and two eyes. "It does look like a cat," says my urologist, looking up at me and smiling. What I came up with next sent us three into volleys of laughter. "Yes," I said, "Stanley's little *pussy.*"

Surely, the doctor's staff must have wondered why it was so funny that he had called me in to tell me I have cancer as I am sure some of them must have heard our gales of laughter outside our examining room. Here is a copy of that slide with my notes and arrows in white.

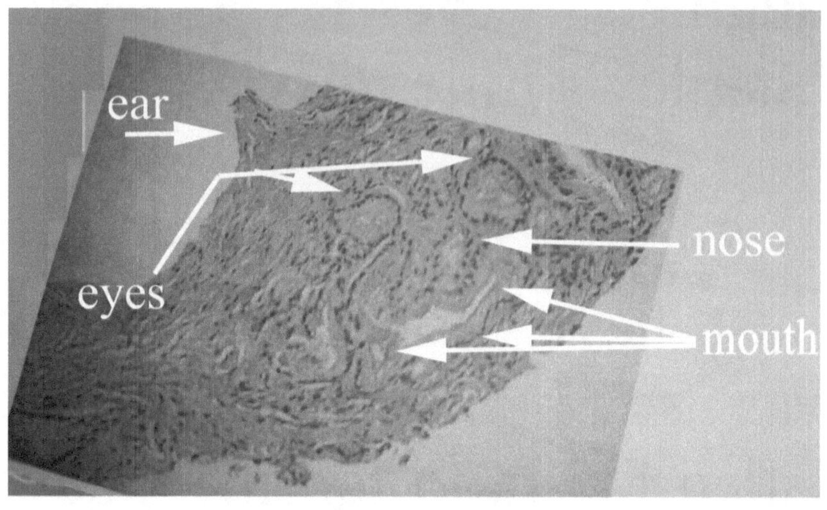


After we stopped laughing, my Doctor said how relieved he was that I found humor in this diagnosis. He told us that some wives begin to cry, some men become indignant and/or incredulous and demand a second opinion and here we were laughing about it. Yes I am sure it could be taken as devastating by lots of people.

Surely enough, here was proof that I had developed an adenocarcinoma. It is defined as a malignant tumor originating in glandular epithelium. My doctor told me not to worry about it, that it was the type of cancer that would grow so slowly that I'd have to live to be 100 years old or more before this tumor would become a threat to my life or health.

As we headed home a book I had read a couple of months before came to mind. I had read it at the urging of my daughter Sheri. The book is THE CHINA STUDY, by T. Colin Campbell, Ph.D. and his son Thomas Campbell II, M.D. The book isn't named well, because it's not a study of just China, but a huge compilation of the diets of peoples from <u>many different</u>

<u>areas in the world,</u> and in addition to their diets, the book reports on their varied levels of wellness and the illnesses which are prevalent in their societies. In fact, it is the most comprehensive worldwide diet/health study of its kind ever done!

This father and son doctor/author team points out that the United States of America leads the world in diabetes, heart disease and of course, the big C, cancer.

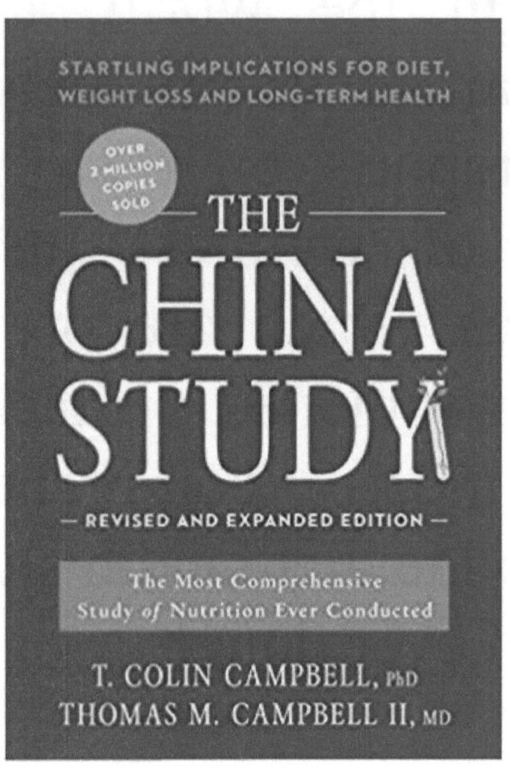


One may conclude it's our diet. Here in the USA lots of animal-based foods are consumed. Is it the animal-based foods that give us a bad time? Well, yes, in part, but

our meats are so laden with problematic chemicals, that those meats are banned from import into the nations of the European Union. The chemicals of which I speak are (1) fertilizers that fertilize the plants on which the animals we eat feed. In addition, we spray our crops with toxic
(2) insecticides and
some possibly carcinogenic
(3) herbicides. This keeps insects from eating our crops

and the herbicides protect our crop fields from weeds.

I once asked a farmer friend, "How come there are no weeds in the cornfield?" "We spray it with RoundUp," was the answer.

As I sit here typing away to compose this book I switched to a search engine to look up subjects like "RoundUp cancer" and found a class action lawsuit internet page offering people who dealt with RoundUp and later found themselves with non-Hodgkin's Lymphoma to contact the sponsoring law firm.

In addition to fertilizers insecticides and herbicides, we find (4) growth hormones, (5) antibiotics and now lately, a chicken grower was cited for administering
(6) tranquilizers to his flock.

Worse, the Huffington Post reported in June of 2012 something of which I'd never heard. It was that traces of the Arsenic compound (7) Roxarsone, a proven carcinogen, were showing up in chicken sold for human consumption. The Huffington Post lamented, "Yet, in June 2011, the FDA gave Pfizer 30 days to discontinue selling Roxarsone, a proven carcinogen. So why is it still showing up in our chickens?"

There's much much more scary stuff in that article and in addition to quoting from it,

I shall furnish you with an internet link that will lead you to the entire article:

**https://www.huffingtonpost.com/ richard-schiffman/antibiotics- chicken_b_1461058.html**

# CHAPTER TWO

## My psychic daughter, is she really?

As it was with my dear late mother, oftentimes I'll go pick up the phone to call my daughter, only to have it ring before I was able to start dialing, and who'd be on the other end? It would be my daughter Sheri who had dialed me up just a few seconds before I got to call her. Conversely, I might ring Sheri on the phone and upon answering she tells me, "I was just going to call you."

When Sheri was five years old she used to dial long distance to call me in spite of her mother's and step-dad's admonition not to call me so much because her calls were generating a lot of toll charges, since she lived in a city a considerable distance from my own. Finally they banned Sheri from calling me altogether. Yet one day Sheri phoned me in spite of the ban.

I answered and when Sheri began to speak, I asked if her long distance calling ban were lifted. "No daddy," she replied, "but I think you are going to do something bad, and I want to tell you 'don't do it.'" In my reply I was less than honest, for I told her, "Well I promise you I won't do anything at bad at all any time ever, ok?" Sheri agreed and we chatted for another minute or so and hung up.

"That kid is psychic," I thought. Well, truth be told, I had just come home in a loaner car from Don Sanderson Ford in Glendale, Arizona, where my new company car was in for its first service. Just before I got that new company car, I received a letter from my then employer, American Can Company with information from Peterson, Howell &

Heather, our company car fleet administrators. I was to choose the make of car, the color, and if I wanted a radio I'd have to pay $35.00 extra. I filled out the form and returned it with a check for the radio. When I picked up my new car, a 1968 four door Ford sedan, it had no radio.

As I sat alone in my house, eating my lunch, I had the thought to **(ALTHOUGH I WOULD NEVER HAVE ACTUALLY DONE IT)** to steal the radio out of the loaner car.....claim it was done in a parking lot.....and then later install it in my company car.

As the thought dissolved, the phone rang. It was little Sheri who had picked up the thought and was calling me to instruct me not to do anything bad, as I wrote a moment ago.

I've always thought there's something to psychic phenomena. I recall reading in

Reader's Digest, a short story about such psychic events.

The event that stuck with me was about two British women, identical twins, born and raised in England. One married an American soldier just as the second world war ended, and settled in the USA with him. A few years later the American sister was involved in a seriously injurious auto accident. At the very moment of the accident, her twin, asleep in her bed in

England, awoke screaming. The article, I recall, finished the tale that although she was seriously injured, the lady survived her injuries with no long-lasting effects.

So now why have I gone on about psychic phenomena and the psychic bond I feel I have with my daughter Sheri? It was that about two months before I was diagnosed with the adenocarcinoma, that Sheri telephoned me here in my Mesa, Arizona home from her home in Morrison, Colorado to tell me, "Dad I just read a book a nurse friend told me about. It's called THE CHINA STUDY, and you've just got to read it. Well I am not, I should not admit, much on book reading, but most often, Sheri's wishes are my commands. So I bought the book and dove in and read it.

On the way home from my urologist's office, when THE CHINA STUDY came to mind, I thought of the Drs.'

Campbell's conclusions that if one were to avoid animal-based foods and just eat plant-based foods, her or his diet would give her or him a greater immune factor and lessen our American diet's high risks of developing (more in my case) cancer, and of course heart disease and diabetes, which my father and his mother both had. My dad took pills and watched his diet, while his overweight mother treated her diabetes with injections of insulin.

The very next day I found myself at my gym, Anytime Fitness. I go there every other day for a workout which includes 30 minutes on an elliptical trainer (a great machine for it "runs" the arms as well as working the legs) followed by a routing of eight weight training machines.

While there, I struck up a conversation with a chap who was at my gym just for the day. He was a professor at a school of medicine in Utah and was in town visiting the family of one of his children. I told him about my diagnosis the day before and how I was considering going on a Vegan diet. He told me I should read EAT TO LIVE, by Joel Fuhrman, M.D. He said that Fuhrman's book was more recently written and was more up to date than THE CHINA STUDY which at that time was fourteen years old.

Interesting that fate would have it that this college

professor from another city would be there at my gym, and further, fate put us together and on the subject of diet and wellness resulting in my learning of Doctor Fuhrman's book.

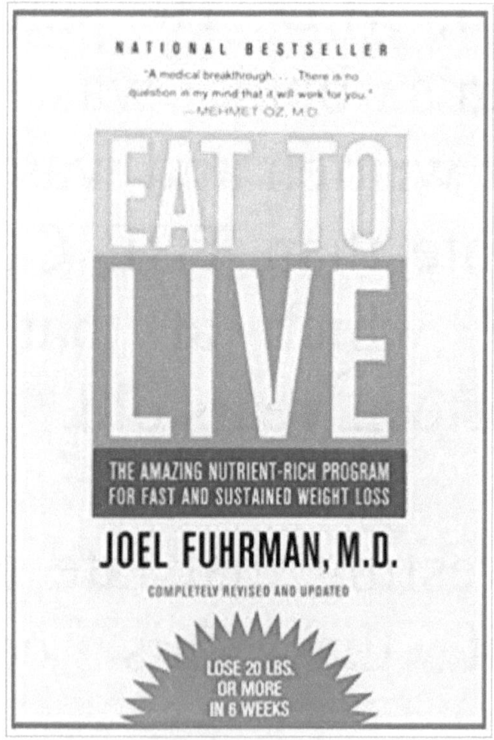

So it was that I got on the internet and ordered a copy of EAT TO LIVE. Fuhrman spends a good bit of the first part admonishing his readers to abandon meat and other animal-based foods. Mind you, this includes milk and milk products, such as cheese, creamy salad dressings, butter, pasta made with milk (many pastas don't incorporate milk these days), baked goods with milk, cream, cheese, whey etc. as an ingredient, including cheesy potato chips, powdered coffee creamers (many say "non-dairy" although some contain *sodium caseinate*, which is a milk product). Casein is a milk product and is found in cheese. Cheese is a very intense, heavily concentrated form of milk product. Casein, according to THE CHINA STUDY, is known to cause kidney damage and is known to promote cancer. Thus cheese, being a concentrated form of milk is the most dangerous form of milk by-product to consume, I've read.

As in beef, the milk that comes from cows contains some of those chemicals we find in the beef that we eat. I won't go on about why Vegans avoid milk and milk by-products. My mission in writing this book doesn't include lecturing on the evils of milk or what some consider a wrongful slaughter of animals so that humans can eat the carcass. That, again, is a subject you can research on the internet and find plenty of information on the topic already written and published by many, many authors.

I will conclude by saying that we are probably one of the least food-supply-protected countries among other similarly advanced nations because those who make our laws are often beholden to others who fund their elections and those financiers and/or their employers will profit financially if their candidate is elected to office as promised by the candidate. I once read that "our Congress is little more than a forum for legalized bribery." This is not to take away from our US Food and Drug Administration which does as good a job as it can, considering the constraints placed upon it.

Did my daughter Sheri have some inkling that I had a

form of cancer (my doctor said it was probably present two months before my diagnosis) and that I might benefit from implementing the diet that reading THE CHINA STUDY would suggest to a cancer victim? No, I can't PROVE that Sheri is psychic because it might be just a coincidence that she recommended that valuable-to-me book.

Psychic or not, THE CHINA STUDY would have

in it the information that I could use to change my diet and either slow or stop my cancer from worsening. Indeed a Vegan diet would serve to help my kidney function numbers, which I learned when going over my laboratory results with my primary healthcare provider.

As well, the Vegan diet helps me stay away from getting diabetes, which, as I said, both my father and his mother had. Finally, the Vegan diet would eventually make me ***heart-attack proof*** according to Dr. Joel Fuhrman's book, EAT TO LIVE.

In my time thinking about changing over to a Vegan diet, I came across a study reported on by The National Institutes of Health (NIH) which concluded in part that the blood serum of Vegans had eight times (800%) more cancer cell killing power than the blood serum of the control group which ate the Standard American Diet (SAD, an appropriate acronym, the author opines). Here is the internet link to the NIH report: (a portion of which is seen next)

**https://www.ncbi.nlm.nih.gov/pubmed/16094059**

*The growth of LNCaP prostate cancer cells (American Type Culture Collection, Manassas, Virginia) was inhibited almost 8 times more by* *serum from the experimental than from the control group (70% vs 9%, p <0.001). Changes in serum PSA and also in LNCaP cell growth were significantly associated with the degree of change in diet and lifestyle.*

***CONCLUSIONS:*** *Intensive lifestyle changes may affect the progression of early, low grade prostate cancer in men.*

*Further studies and longer term followup are warranted.*

You can dig up the information on this blood serum/cancer cell killing information by searching on the internet with the phrase, *"vegans have eight times the cancer cell killing characteristics."*

# CHAPTER THREE
## THE IMPORTANCE OF EXERCISE

This would be a good time to talk about exercise, since in chapter two I mentioned my gym as the spot where I met the professor from Utah.

I am ALL ABOUT EXERCISE. I once read that the human body was meant to work and work hard.

In designing machines to do much of our work, we deny our bodies what they crave, and that's hard work.

You will read here and there that endorphins are among the chemicals that can be generated in the brain which function to transmit electrical signals along our bodies' neuropathways. Endorphins can work to reduce our perceptions of pain, but more important to you and me, they generate a positive feeling in the body and brain. Many is the time that I headed to the gym, wishing I could just turn around and go do something else, but I have made a strong personal bond with the habit of overcoming that negative thought process and gone ahead and finished a full workout at which time I feel all pepped up, happy, and full of self-congratulations on having stayed with it to get my rewards.

***As well, anything you work to establish as constant repetitive behavior*** to move from bad stuff (like smoking cigarettes) to good stuff, like persisting in always wanting to learn new things or forcing yourself to drive safely in a successful effort to avoid the temptation to step up the speed to get there more quickly, ***becomes indelibly part of your habitual behavioral package***. You will feel as compelled to get to the gym or wherever you do your exercises as the smoker feels compelled to pull out a cigarette and light up. <u>Repetitive behavior is very addictive. Use it to your benefit!</u>

So I can't think of anything better I would recommend to you, cancer patient or not, than to adopt a good, worthwhile program of exercise. If you are over forty years of age it is recommended that you have a cardiologist clear you to begin a new program.

If you are not sure of what you'd like to do, visit a gymnasium and engage the personal trainer there. She or he will guide you individually to a wise, meaningful program of physical fitness.

When I was about forty years of age I dug a hole in my back yard to accommodate a cement base on which I subsequently mounted a 71 foot Amateur Radio tower. The hole was three feet wide on all four sides, and six feet deep. I dug out two cubic yards of dirt over a weekend and on the following Monday morning I awoke with severe back pain. I had badly strained my back. My doctor sent me home from work with instructions to take my muscle relaxers and lounge around like a couch potato for two weeks.

When I reported back to my doctor at the end of two

weeks, he asked me if I'd consider guided exercise to strengthen myself up in all quarters. "If you don't," he cautioned me, "You'll hurt yourself as you did two weeks ago every time you do something that strenuous."

I told him I was interested and he told me about a retired Marine who ran an exercise program about a mile away at the downtown YMCA in Phoenix. I enrolled in a three-day-a-week program which began just a half hour after work. On my first day I stopped and leaned against the wall in utter fatigue, trying to catch my breath, and this was just from doing the warm-ups.

In the months that followed I lost about 20 pounds of *blubber* and in about two weeks, I could keep up with the rest of my fellow gymrats.

Ever since that time I have worked out with exercise

equipment in my own home gym or gone to a public gym such as the Anytime Fitness here in east Mesa, Arizona, to which I belong at no charge these days (it's paid for by my Medicare Advantage health-care program).

So in my forties I renewed my body to one in which I still feel pride. My wife and I began to go running and we found ourselves competing in 10K (a race over a ten kilometer/6.6 mile course) events and we found skiing at high altitudes no problem whatsoever. Today I am 82 years old and as you know, still a "gymrat."

# CHAPTER FOUR
## THE DECISION TO GO VEGAN

So I began to research that which it is I must eat to maximize my intake of nutritious foods. I didn't want to just eat *anything* that wasn't meat or eggs or fish or milk (animal-based foods) or any of its by-products. What I Did want to do was to find out what were the MOST NUTRITIOUS FOODS available and just eat those!

One document I found worth much was **Eleven Things Healthy Vegans Eat**. I shall include a link to it below. What I want to stress is that after I learned what the most nutritious foods were, I determined on my own that I must switch from one food to another, to avoid the peril of ignoring some nutrients and concentrating on just a few. In short, I wanted **the greatest variety of the strongest nutrients** I could ingest.

The link to the article of the eleven things is here: https://www.healthline.com/ nutrition/foods-vegans- eat#section1

I urge you to use the link and read all the supporting text to each of the eleven foods, rather  than just depend on the list as follows.

Those foods, briefly, are:
1-LEGUMES
2-NUTS, NUT BUTTERS AND SEEDS
3-HEMP, FLAX AND CHIA SEEDS
4-TOFU AND OTHER MINIMALLY PROCESS-ED MEAT SUBSTITUTES
5-CALCIUM-FORTIFIED PLANT MILKS & YOGURTS
6-SEAWEED
7-NUTRITIONAL YEAST

# 8-SPROUTED & FERMENTED PLANT FOODS

# 9-WHOLE GRAINS, CEREALS AND PSEUDOCEREALS

# 10-CHOLINE-RICH FOODS

# 11-FRUITS AND VEGETABLES

# CHAPTER FIVE

## FROM DIAGNOSIS TO A NEGATIVE BIOPSY

At this point I would like to submit my timelines for you.

### (1)

It was on February 22, 2016 that I received news that I had adenocarcinoma of the prostate, which, as I said, is the slow-growing form of prostate cancer, which as I also said earlier, is, as I said my doctor offered, suffered by 80% of 80 year old men in the USA. Most urologists recommend what is called, "watchful waiting." This means that since slow-growing prostate cancer usually takes so long to be lethal, that most men die of other causes. As a result, no treatment is recommended by most urologists.

(2)

On September 7, 2016, an MRI with mild contrast showed a "suggestion," said the cautious radiologist, that the disease had spread (not metastasized) into the vas deferens, outside the prostate itself. This, if indeed it had moved to the vas deferens, would move the growth to a stage three cancer.

## (3)

On October 19, 2017, I had a sight-guided, MRI biopsy of eleven tissue samples done in my urologist's office. The results were that, in not so much as one of those eleven tissue samples, was a cancer cell present! Thus in fifteen months of a Vegan diet, my cancer had disappeared. Needless to say I was jubilant.

# CHAPTER SIX

# "GOING VEGAN?"
## WHY IS THIS SO SCARY?

In the years during which I practiced psychology, my flagship offering was behavior therapy and hypnosis for weight loss. It was a good way to keep a full appointment schedule in that market of then just 60,000 souls (Mesa County Colorado, which includes the city of

Grand Junction). I would say that the overweight people who came to me and were successful with their weight losses, had already gotten themselves psychologically prepared for change and were ready to do what it took to lose that extra weight. That *self-preparation* is what, I believe, made them so accepting of the idea of altering their eating habits, which they and I worked together to achieve.

So when I would explain to family and friends how I altered my diet to avoid animal-based foods, I was taken aback at how most manifested body language and verbal comments were of UTTER REVULSION.

At first I was almost as freaked out at their repugnance as they were freaked out at the idea of like dropping hamburgers, steak, milk, ice cream and other animal-based foods.

I put thought into this behavior and came to the conclusion that indeed, very many people are more in love with their eating habits than they are concerned about mounting an all-out fight against their cancer or eating to avoid cancer (diabetes and heart disease). A friend who's had breast cancer told me, "I just couldn't do it." She added that she admired my will power.

For me it was a no-brainer that I needed to avoid foods that were, first, not very nutritious, but more important, second, contained those chemicals mentioned earlier that were KNOWN CARCINOGENS. "Who in their right mind, would eat these **known** carcinogens?" I puzzled.

Well obviously, not all of us are alike. As you know, some people are tied inextricably to their habitual behaviors, and others can walk away from a bad habit in a heartbeat. The difference would be whether or not a person had a strong sense of self-preservation coupled with the ability to make a decision for evading toxins in his or her diet and sticking to it and the degree that their personality had to accept change. At one end of the spectrum are those who readily embrace change and at the other, those who fight change, with endless variations in between.

I am among those who doesn't care what he or she eats. I am like, well I could just as well end up at a Burger King or McDonald's in Europe to grab a quick lunch as a fine restaurant.

Yet a traveling companion who loved cooking and delighted in gourmet cooking and was eager to learn about foods in distant lands, might tell me, were I to suggest lunch at "that Burger King over there," "If you think I am going to eat in a Burger King in Paris, France, you have another think coming." That actually happened to me once in Paris. The one who said that was my now wife of fifteen years, Marlene.

## MAKING THE CHANGE

vegnews.com reported in September of 2018 that Vegan food sales had spiked to 3.7 billion dollars during a twelve month period. They estimate that it is headed to be a ten billion dollar industry in the near future. So Vegan eating is on the rise. I once read that an acre of land can feed many more people if plants for human consumption are raised on it, than if it were set up as pasture for animals to be killed and eaten by humans.

If you want to begin exploring the idea of basing your Vegan diet considerations on inhumane behavior, consider the following that I found on sentientmedia.org: *"More than 200 million animals are killed for food around the world every day – just on land. That comes out to 72 billion land animals killed for food around the world every year. Including wild caught and farmed fishes, we get a daily total closer to 3 billion animals killed."*

Anyway, what helped me very much in giving up animal based foods was the fact that there are what I consider *"transition foods."* Transition foods, as I call them, are those that helped me move away from meat and dairy. I found some stores that have joined the slow but sure movement among grocers to begin to add Vegan items to their stock. In January of 2020 my wife Marlene came home from a shopping foray quite excitedly anxious to tell me that our local COSTCO had just established a quite sizeable Vegan foods section! BRAVO COSTCO!

Right now I really enjoy eating the imitation meat and

imitation "transition foods," as I call them. I can not yet say that the day will come when I will move away from them. Indeed, like old helpful friends, I might keep loving them and keep them around, although they are more costly than the non-Vegan similar meats, cheeses, etc. Time will tell.

As it is now I use these transition foods fairly often in working as hard as I can to keep a rotating variety of nutrients in my diet.

Here are some of my favorite "transition foods:" Lightlife Mexican crumbles & Daiya cheese substitutes.

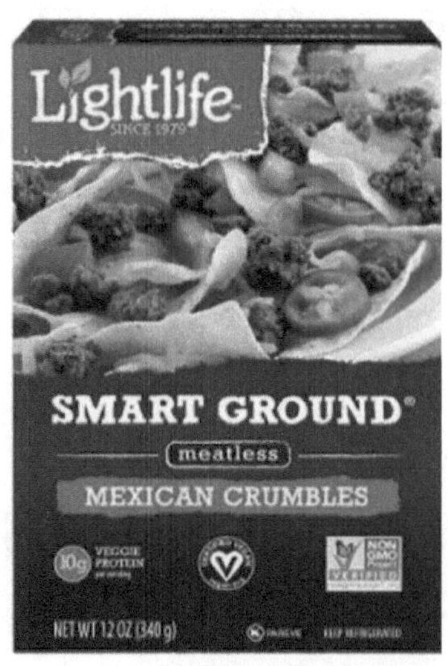
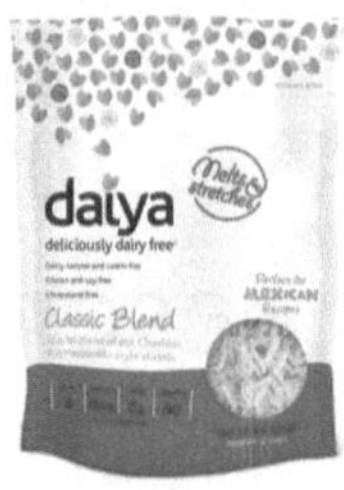
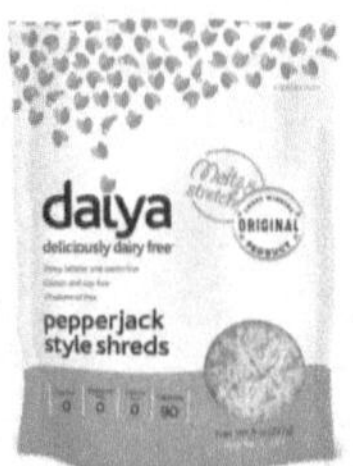
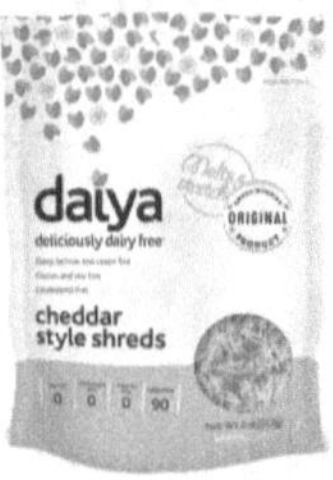
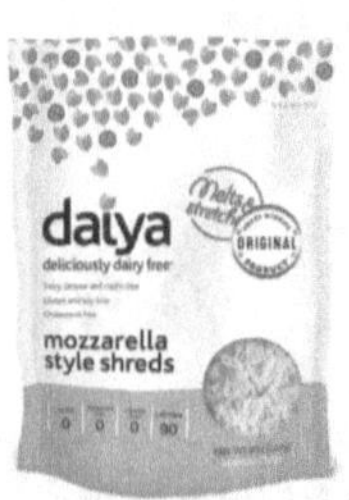

If you go to an up-to-date grocer and find these items in

the refrigerated case, then you should find other foods by Lightlife and Daiya plus other transitional foods. If you visit the frozen section you can find delightfully meat-tasting veggie burgers, or fake sausage patties, both made by Morningstar Farms. One Morningstar product I absolutely love is their Buffalo (breaded) Chik Patties. They are also available in a less spicy version as Original Chik

Patties. Here's a picture of the Buffalo Chik version;

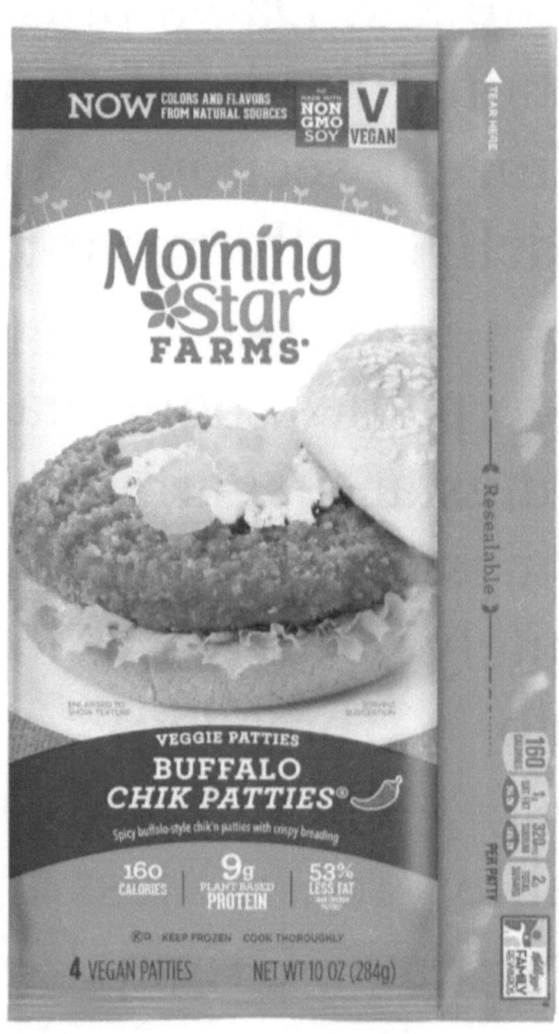

I must make mention of a warning; a Morningstar Farms telephone representative told me in 2019 that sometime in 2020 all Morningstar Farms products will be 100% Vegan. Right now the Chik Patties are, but the Morningstar Spicy Black Bean patties are not. Read the ingredients from time to time to see if Morningstar has transitioned to fully Vegan products.

# Um….well Stan, what about dessert???

I gotcha' covered friend! There ARE "transition" foods for dessert and the ones that pop into my mind first and foremost are the various flavors of Ben & Jerry's non-dairy desserts. I personally feel that they taste EVERY BIT AS GOOD AS DAIRY-BASED ICE CREAM!

My two favorites are Cherry Garcia and Cinnamon Buns. There are some new ones out now (May 3, 2019) that I have yet to try and my grocery store is hard put to carry the full line. I will paste some photos in here for you to peruse.  At the end of my book is my email address and I invite you to let me know how you find those items.  Here is a url to visit: https://www.benjerry.com/about-us/contact-us

When you get there you can click *Where can I find my favorite flavor?*  Then you click the Flavor Locator and enter your zip code.  Here are four photos that include my two favorite flavors, Cherry Garcia and Cinnamon Buns and a couple of others I'd like to try.

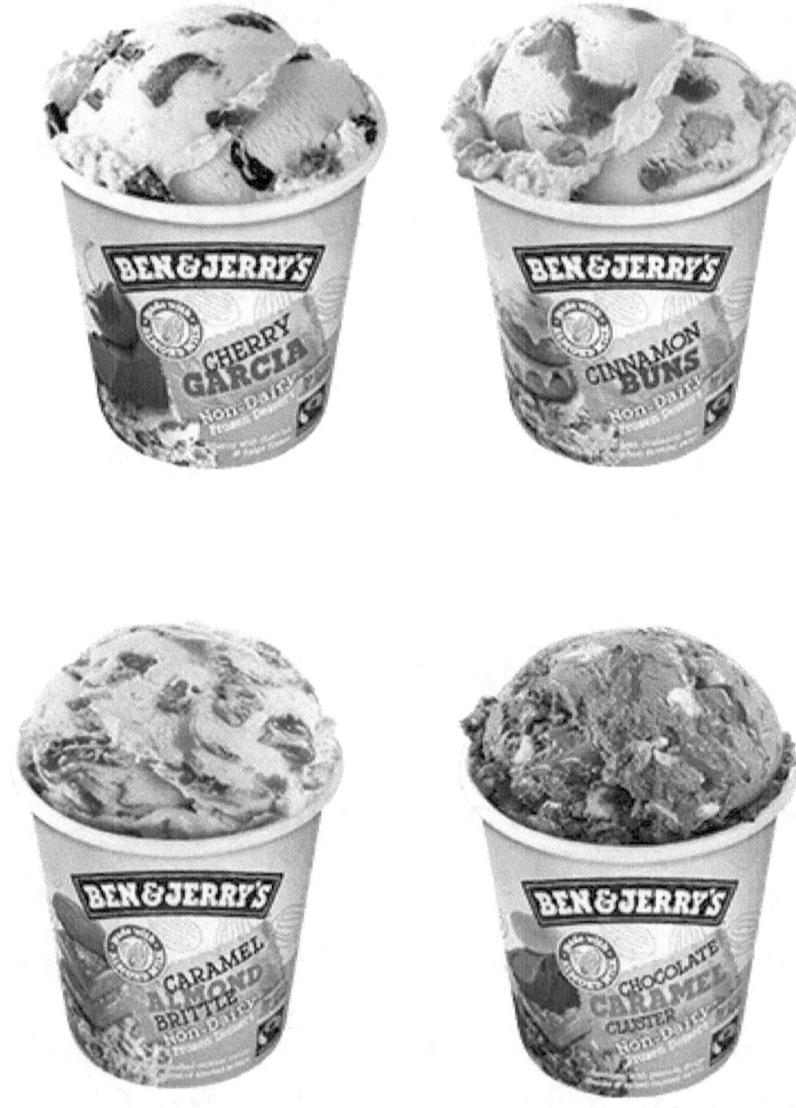
BEN&JERRY'S
CHERRY
GARCIA
Non-Dairy
BEN&JERRY'S
CINNAMON
BUNS
Non-Dairy
BEN&JERRY'S
CARAMEL
ALMOND
BRITTLE
Non-Dairy
BEN&JERRY'S
CHOCOLATE
CARAMEL
CLUSTER
Non-Dairy

# CHAPTER SEVEN

## THE HEALING POWER OF THE HUMAN BRAIN

Way back in the early 1980s, when I was practicing psychology in Grand Junction, Colorado, I attended a seminar called THE HEALING POWER OF THE HUMAN BRAIN.

I would not have attended had not one of my heroes

been scheduled to do a presentation there, but he was there and was a presenter. One of my heroes? Yes, he was part of a two-person hero combination. The second person of this combination was his then-wife.

The man of whom I speak is the late O. Carl Simonton, M.D., a radiation oncologist. His then-wife was Stephanie Matthews Simonton, described here and there on the internet these days as a

"Psychotherapist." I could not find anything about Ms. Matthews' college education or any degrees she might hold.

That said, between this man and wife oncologist-psychotherapist team, it was discovered that cancer victims, or patients, if you will, had certain personality traits in common. One of them was altruism.

I find altruism best defined as acts of promoting the welfare of another person, no matter the risk or cost to the altruist. In my readings and experience I have discovered this stark reality, put boldly here: If you don't do first for yourself, nature will take a dim view of you and your lack of self-interest and self-promotion and will undermine the strength of your immune system. It is as if nature wants to "take out" those who don't do for themselves primarily. It seems ***YOU NEED A SENSE OF STRONG SELF-PURPOSE*** to keep your immune system operating at maximum strength.

The Simontons also discovered that many cancers manifest themselves within one year of a very upsetting, adverse event in the victim's life. This might include divorce, the death of a spouse or child, being imprisoned, getting fired, among many other very adverse life events.

You might do well to read Simontons' book, GETTING WELL AGAIN, which explains all of this and much more in scholarly detail.

I must add here that Dr. Simonton choked on a piece of food while eating a meal in his Agoura Hills, California home in July of 2009 which sadly caused his death at sixty six years of age.

GETTING WELL AGAIN ISBN-9780963293466, was originally published in 1978 by St. Martin's Press and is easily found to this day where books are sold.

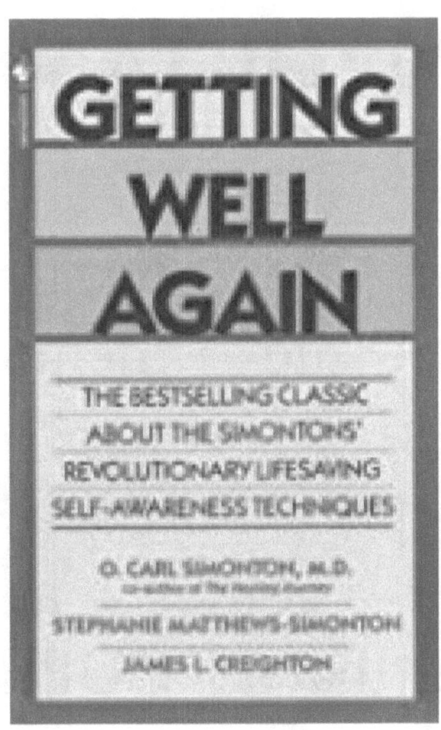

# CHAPTER EIGHT

## TOMATOES ARE IMPORTANT!

I can't let you get away without the mention of tomatoes! From Spain's Universitat Politècnica de València comes a study showing that LYCOPENE, an antioxidant found in tomatoes, which gives tomatoes their red color, is a strong protector against cancer, in particular, prostate cancer. In that report, a bowl of tomato sauce is shown next to a serving of French-fried potatoes. Here's a link to am article about that Spanish study: **http://tinyurl.com/y4qwtjwj**

**BEFORE I SAY ANOTHER WORD I WANT YOU TO KNOW THAT LYCOPENE IN PILLS, CAPSULES OR WHAT-HAVE-YOU IS**

## **TOTALLY WORTHLESS! This is per yet another study I read on the subject.**

I read of a study of elderly men with prostate cancer on a special diet to track their diet vs. cancer progress. The men were "drinking tomato <u>sauce</u>."

Okay, I drink tomato sauce every morning in diluted form. I buy 64 ounce bottles of Walmart's private label copy of V8 vegetable juice or sometimes Walmart's tomato juice (see photo below for Walmart's vegetable juice) and I mix up a brew consisting of about 35% vegetable or tomato juice and 65% tomato sauce. Then I shake it up, stick it in the fridge and drink a glass of it every morning with breakfast! Sometimes, not often, I just drink a can of tomato sauce with breakfast! Have a look at the photos of these drinks on the next page:

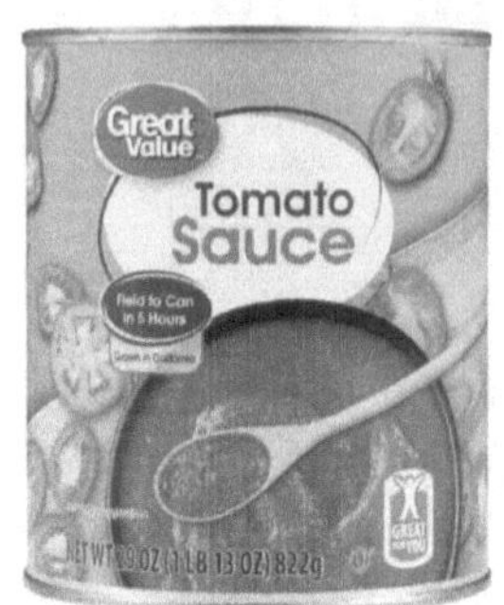

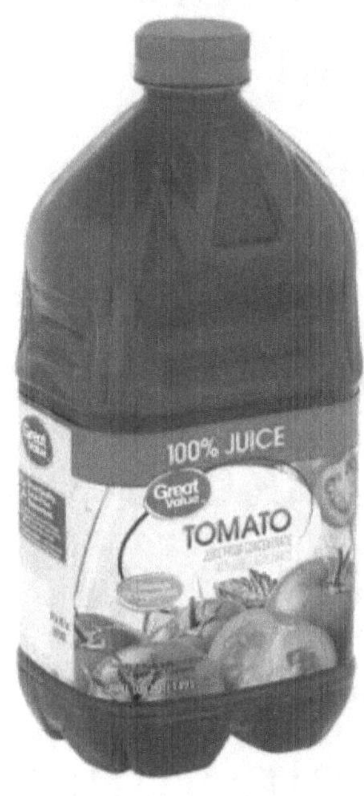

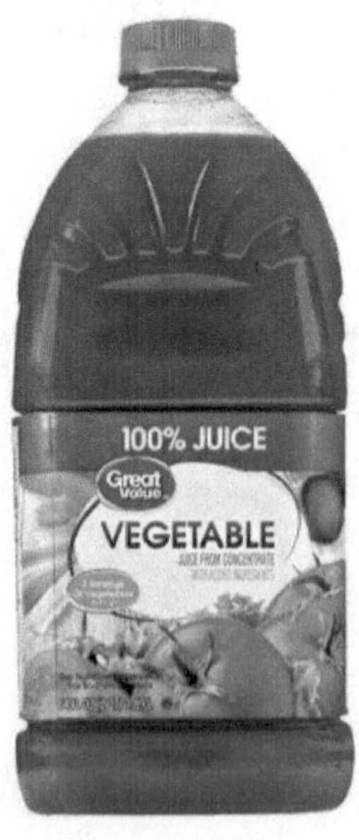

# CHAPTER NINE
# A WORD OF CAUTION

I am writing this chapter because I am aware of people who "beat cancer" by using methods alternative to those suggested by their medical doctor physician/s. If you opt not to go the route of radiation and chemotherapy if suggested by your doctor, then it's at your risk. I can't recommend failing to take advice from a licensed, board certified physician, although you may opt to do that. It's your body, it's your future, it's your call. Maybe get a second opinion!

I recall the movie actor Steve McQueen was stricken with mesothelioma, an incurable cancer of the lungs that can develop due to exposure to asbestos. It was thought that McQueen's car racing suits, which were filled with asbestos to resist exposure to fire, were responsible for McQueen's disease. McQueen dropped traditional American therapies and went to Mexico in July of 1980 to undergo a mixture of what have been since proven to be worthless therapies.

McQueen, with the help of American and Mexican doctors, followed a plan designed by a Doctor William D. Kelley, an American orthodontist who claimed his concoction of therapies cured his own pancreatic cancer.

McQueen subjected himself to Kelley's package of therapies which were as follows: take pancreatic enzymes, ingest 50 vitamin and mineral dosages every day, receive massages, take coffee enemas, attend prayer sessions, undergo psychotherapy, undergo injections of a cell preparation made up of cattle and sheep fetuses, and take Laetrile, a substance derived from apricot pits which has never proven to be effective against cancer.

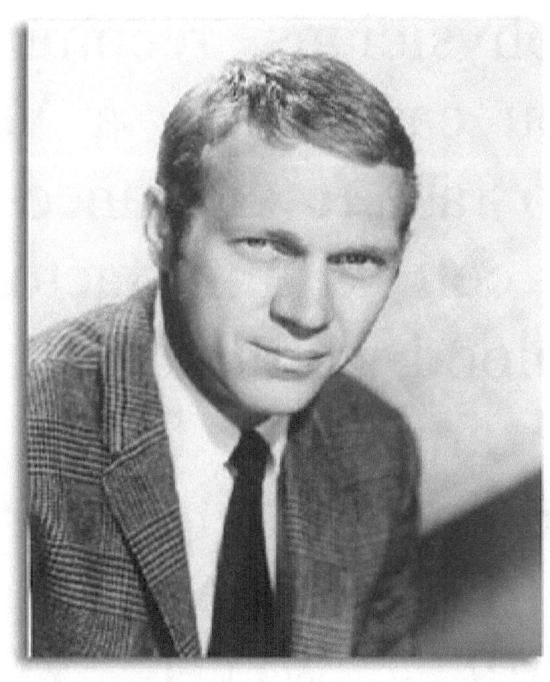

Steve McQueen

McQueen had surgery the following November to remove some cancerous masses. He passed away the day after the surgery. Moral of the story: stay with what your physicians recommend and you can follow a Vegan diet so as to enhance the cancer cell killing factor of your blood serum. You can also do any other things you fancy doing to help yourself, BUT LET THEM BE IN CONCERT WITH YOUR PHYSICIAN'S

# RECOMMENDED TREATMENT AND WITH HER OR HIS APPROVAL.

My cancer was, as I've said here, the slow-growing prostate cancer that is treated by what many doctors call, "watchful waiting." As was said before here, I was told that 80 percent of us 80 year old American men have this cancer and that my cancer was not life threatening. So I was offered neither radiation nor chemotherapy. However, if I had aggressive cancer, I'd certainly have followed my physician's recommendation for treatment, including radiation and/or chemo-therapy.

Concurrent with that which I've said heretofore, my advice on changing your diet to avoid animal-based foods would be to use it as an **_augment_** to your medical treatment,

# EMPHATICALLY NOT IN PLACE OF IT!
# Just BEWARE! OKAY?

All this said, I had a man tell me during his fight with cancer that his doctor told him to eat a lot of meat to obtain protein. EARTH TO THAT DOCTOR! Hello! *There is plenty of protein in plant-based foods. Look up the protein content of any of the plant-based foods, AND read the protein grams on labels of cans of plant-based foods, especially beans. You can get your protein from the same source that the animals you ate got protein; PLANTS!*

An article in Popular Science (popsci.com) by Sarah Chodosh published in June of 2018, explained that plant-based protein is much healthier nutritionally (has much more roughage) and more abundant than that found in meat. So that doctor needed a wake-up call! We have a long way to go to change thinking in many corners.

Now then, there are people who will try to sell you this or that treatment or medication, knowing fully that what they have to offer is a hoax, and on the other hand, there are those who will solicit you to spend your money with them, fully and sincerely believing that what they have to offer will actually help you fight your cancer, but it won't. They are among those of us in society who believe in falsehoods. I would compare them to those who believe that the vapor trail that appears behind a high-flying jet airplane is not water vapor, but a toxic gas (they call them "chemtrails") that some entity is dispersing into our atmosphere to do this or that to us. Their beliefs are borne on the wings of less than healthy minds. Indeed those sorts of people are paranoid to one degree of another and certainly they are void of any sense of intellectual curiosity!

Next, I urge you to evade at all costs, anyone who tells you that a lot of, or even MOST physicians won't tell you those things that will cure you, so that they can keep you coming to them to spend more of your money with them. They will tell you that the pharmaceutical industry is doing the same thing to you, that is, offering you medications that are not going to cure you, so that you will continue to buy those medications so as to assure a continuous stream of income for that *less-than-honest* (they will tell you) pharmaceutical industry.

I assert that these conspiracy nutcases are another gaggle of sick or dishonest, or both, people who will, wittingly or unwittingly block your path to wellness.

# I COULD NOT MORE STRONGLY RECOMMEND THAT IN ADDITION TO ALTERING YOUR DIET, THAT YOU WORK WITH A LICENSED UROLOGIST, OR LICENSED ONCOLOGIST TO UNDERGO WHAT SHE OR HE RECOMMENDS IN THE WAY OF ANY MEDICATION, RADIATION, AND CHEMOTHERAPY!

# CHAPTER TEN
## THANK YOU AND GOODBYE

Thank you for having purchased and read this little book. I purposely kept it free of fluffy stuffing for the sole purpose of making it bigger than it needed to be. *"GET TO THE POINT"* is what I am all about.

For now, my cancer's gone. As you know, my cancer was the non-aggressive, slow-growing version of prostate cancer, which, as I've also said here, multiple times (yes I know, LOL) is not life-threatening.

Most of us guys with this type of cancer die of other causes before our particular type of cancer could cause our death.

Yes, for now my cancer's gone. It could well reappear one day and oh yes, my urologist and I will keep an eye on it.

Once in a while I will admit, I cheat on my diet. I have a bag of potato chips from Walmart in my cupboard that contain and are flavored with cheese and sour cream. One night a month ago I ate two pieces of regular pizza with dairy cheese and a few pepperoni slices.

I would say that my cheating occurs with a very small item and no more than two or three times a year. My wife Marlene is amazed at my self-control as are some of our friends.

To others who see what I am eating and question me, I explain that I am not a Vegan because I abhor the slaughter of animals, although I am slowly finding myself more and more thinking what an inhumane thing it is to murder an animal since I went Vegan, that such cruel and bloody slaughter takes place.

I explain that my Vegan diet reduced what was described as a stage 3 cancer with an MRI narrative report suggesting a spread of the disease into the Vas Defrens, and that in fifteen months, my eating only plant-based foods is that to which I ascribe the complete disappearance of my cancer that was discovered on October 19, 2017.

Should you like to contact me, you may email me at stan.rocklin@gmail.com

Thank you again, and goodbye.

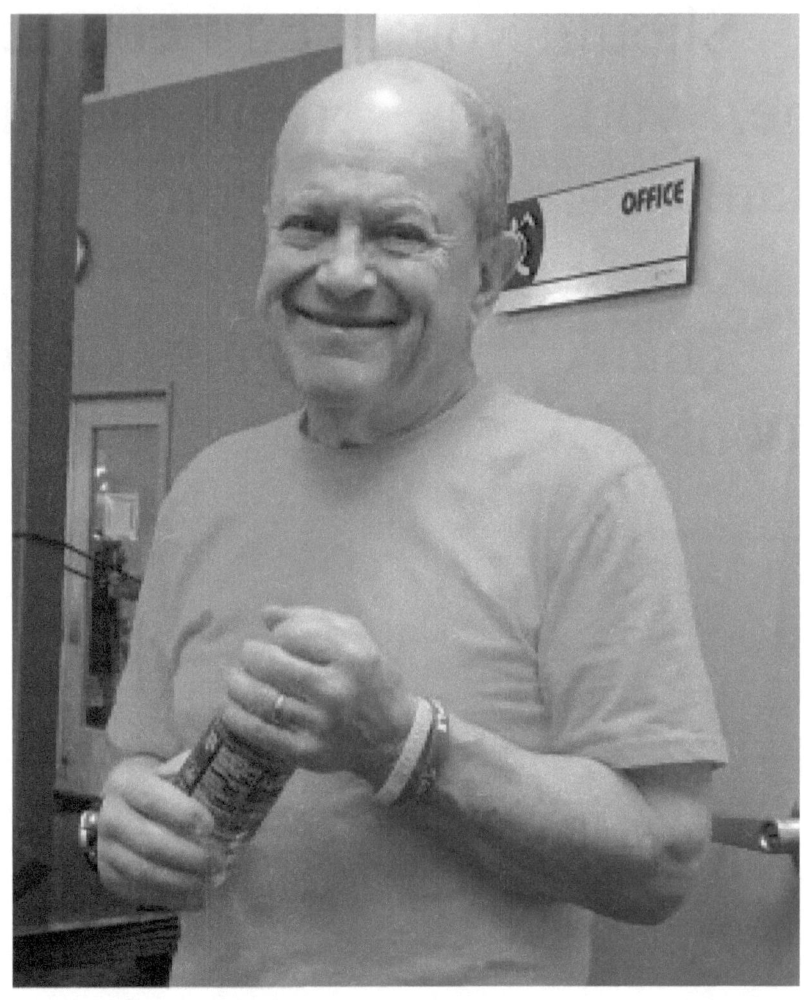

The author at his gym, Anytime Fitness,
8257 E. Guadalupe Rd., Mesa, AZ